The Physique Formula
Unlocking The Human Performance
Edge

Jimmy Smith,MS,CSCS
For Exclusive Content Visit
http://www.physiqueformuladiet.com

Disclaimer

No part of this publication may be reproduced, transmitted, transcribed, stored in a retrieval system, or translated into any language in any form, by any means, without the written permission of the author.

The information contained within this guide and the associated files in this folder is for informational purposes only and includes our communications over phone, text messages, emails, facebook, twitter and youtube and it is intended for your use only.

It is not the intention of Jimmy Smith Training LLC or Jimmy Smith to provide specific medical advice or diagnosis, but rather to provide the user with information to better understand their health and fitness.

This information is only intended for your personal use.

There are inherent health risks associated with any physical activity. By continuing to work with Jimmy Smith Training, LLC, you acknowledge their risks and voluntarily assume any and all risk of loss, damage, or injury that may result including personal injury, accidents or illness, including death.

About The Author

Jimmy Smith,MS,CSCS is a recognized leader in the field of human performance and offers a unique blend of cutting edge nutrition and training information to his elite athletes and clients. As a writer, speaker and coach, Jimmy has helped professional and elite athletes in 6 different major sports and recreational athletes in over 74 different countries reach a higher level of performance and physique development.

Jimmy has been featured on ESPN Radio, ABC News, CBS Sports and in Men's Fitness and Men's Health magazines and his best selling book, The Physique Formula, and has helped hundreds of athletes and health enthusiasts attain leaner and healthier physiques .

Jimmy is also an athlete himself, having played high level of college basketball, and continues to use himself as a human performance experiment in order to give his athletes the legal and natural edge to become champions.

His website http://www.jimmysmithtraining.com offers consulting, articles, interviews and videos.

He offers daily helpful video at http://www.youtube.com/jimmysmithtraining

You can follow him on twitter at http://www.twitter.com/jimmysmithtrain

You can "Like" his fan page at http://www.facebook.com/physiqueformula

Praise For The Physique Formula

I started working with Jimmy Smith in 2012. I immediately got great information and his coaching made my training and weight loss much easier.

He is a genius. I'm a private coaching client, and that's the only way to go. Having someone there to guide you is priceless.

All the years I killed myself trying to make weight I thought that was the only way. My last couple of mma fights where easier to make weight than any other time in my career. I never felt like I was struggling with the diet either. I get to eat great food and the fat just melts away. Same thing with his water cutting system. Hardly any effort and I make weight with ease. Jimmy has taken me from 212 to 205 in 2 weeks and from 205 to 185 in 2 days and I never felt like I was starving or "dieting". Jimmy is the man, he's the top nutrition expert right now in my opinion.

Dedicated to mma and grappling,
Alan Belcher, MMA middleweight fighter

I would like to give a shout out to the herald of accuracy Jimmy Smith. One of the best mma specific nutritionist out there. Jimmy has helped me make weight multiple times and worked with me in modifying my diets. He is open minded and regardless of what nutritional beliefs you have he can work with you to improve your plan. I would recommend him to anyone I know, no bullshit.

Jake Lindsey, MMA lightweight fighter

My fight was in the 155 division but a month out of the fight my weight was around 167. I spent hours looking for articles online when eventually I came across Jimmy Smith's website and sent him a email. After a few emails I decided to give his 3 day weight cutting program a try. During the 3 days I strictly followed his instructions. I had a 15 hour drive to the event and following his instructions I was able to maintain my energy and make the drive comfortable. Weigh ins also got pushed back two hours. Even with the obstacles I never felt dizzy or lacked energy and always felt my health was in good shape. I weighed in at 155 then followed the instructions of how to refuel and come fight time I had all my weight,strength and energy back. I was able to keep a strong pace in the first round before winning the fight shortly into the second round.

Laine Keyes, MMA lightweight fighter

Just needed to give you a shout out and thank you!

After many years in this fitness journey (starting in 1991) I was ready for some different, fresh ideas to add to my mix of eating skills and you saved the day! I have been reading your emails and updates for months and am so happy I made the decision to give you a holler.

I've been enjoying my 'freedom' from the strict nonsense of eating frequently and feel refreshed and energized with your options for food and simple supplementation. Thank you for tweaking my thoughts and helping me to see some new angles and twists on my nutrition plan!

Monica Brant,1998 IFBB Fitness Olympia Champion,
2010 and 2013 WBFF World's Pro Figure Champion

Table of Contents

Introduction

Anyone can write a meal plan that helps you lose weight, but are you really reaching a higher level of performance? Your goal as an athlete should be to continually progress and get better from workout to workout, month to month and year to year. If that isn't your goal, then you need to think twice about why you're in the sport to begin with because somewhere your future opponent is out-working you.

During my career as a nutritional consultant I have had the great pleasure of working with high level athletes from numerous sports which includes professional hockey, football and golf, United States track and field, college football and track and field, the United States armed forces, and, of course, mixed martial arts.

While the demands of all those sports are drastically different, one parallel exists. All those athletes wanted an advanced nutritional plan drilled down to an easy to follow system. I appreciate science and I am very much on the cutting edge of human performance, but I also understand that not everyone has the same love for the science behind the methods.

If you want more in-depth and detailed information beyond what I present here on elevating testosterone naturally, reducing brain trauma and improving cognitive function and advanced joint repair techniques, then head to the following link below. You'll find all of that information in-depth there.

http://www.physiqueformuladiet.com

What you will find in the following pages is a distilled culmination of my years as a nutritional consultant with elite athletes broken down into a system that you can use today to see noticeable results.

I'd like to extend a special consultation to any athlete that reads this book and wants to learn cutting edge, LEGAL, ways to enhance their performance. Simply email me at jimmy@jimmysmithtraining.com

Expect Greatness!
Jimmy Smith,MS,CSCS
www.jimmysmithtraining.com

The Ten Biggest Nutrition Problems Athletes Face

Before we can get into the actual diet, we first need to address several limiting factors that, unbeknownst to you, have likely been hindering your performance and physique to a significant level for some time.

You have poor insulin management

A lack of insulin sensitivity limits your body's ability to affectively handle, store and use carbohydrates. This leads to fatigue, fat gain, slower muscle growth, poor sleep quality and generally reduced performance. I've seen athletes who feel sluggish and gain fat after eating only one small serving of rice or pasta.

The majority of diets for high level athletes fail because they do not provide adequate amounts of carbohydrates and I've seen this time and time again when an athlete comes to me for the first time. Remember, carbohydrates aren't the enemy. They provide a very efficient energy source for training and can also lead to greater lean muscle growth.

Limiting carbohydrates leads to poor energy levels, impaired sleep patterns, lower natural testosterone, higher levels of the muscle

3

wasting hormone cortisol and increased stress levels.

The goal is to find a sweet spot for carbohydrate intake and this is done by assessing your goals, body fat levels and training activity, among multiple other factors. Just because you train doesn't mean that you should be eating large bowls of pasta every night.

Remember, it's less about what you eat and more about what gets into your cells to fuel performance.

Simple ways to improve your insulin sensitivity

-Limit your starchy carbohydrate intake to your pre and post workout times and possibly a tiny amount before bed.

-Consume 6-9 grams of a high quality Omega-3 fish oil supplement daily.

-Lose body fat until you have visual abdominal definition and aim to stay at that level as long as you can.

You have high cortisol levels

Cortisol is a muscle wasting hormone that when elevated increases body fat levels, reduces testosterone and interrupts cognitive function which leads to monetary confusion, while also causing the body to use muscle tissue for energy. That's something we obviously don't want. High cortisol also leads to nagging and frequent joint pain.

Unfortunately, in today's day and time most athletes actually engage in practices that raise cortisol, including confusing high amounts of stimulants like caffeine, sugary post workout drinks, products containing artificial sweeteners or by just being deficient in essential trace micronutrients

Simple ways to reduce your cortisol levels

-Aim to lower your sugar consumption and if you must, only eat it immediately after your workout.

-Take 1-2 grams of a high quality Vitamin C supplement spread out three to four times per day.

-Reduce your caffeine intake and consider switching from coffee to green tea.

You have adrenal fatigue

This goes hand in hand with high cortisol levels. Your adrenals are small grape sized glands that rest above your kidneys. The role of the adrenal glands is to dictate and control hormone production when the adrenals are fatigued from too much stress, caffeine, sugar or training.

As the adrenals continually get more and more fatigued, the body's hormonal patterns don't operate the way they should. Athletes I work with often complain of waking up tired while having trouble getting to sleep and staying asleep. Another common symptom is muscle soreness that lasts longer than usual.

High performance athletes are hard workers and tend to think that they need to train more and more for longer periods of time. That's a recipe for disaster. Everything needs to be changed when the adrenal glands are fatigued.

Simple ways to recover from adrenal fatigue

-Lower your total training time a few days per week.

-Consider supplementing with a high quality B Vitamin Complex two to three times per day.
- Aim to drink 1-2 cups of green tea per day.

Your body cannot properly absorb nutrients

Following a clean, good diet is only 50% of the battle. Eating nutritious foods is great, but only if your body is absorbing the vitamins and minerals in those foods. The very first thing that I do when I start working with athletes is to help them rebuild their stomach acid. Your stomach produces hydrochloric acid in order to activate digestive enzymes that break down the food you just ate. Unfortunately, stress, artificial sweeteners, too much sugar and starchy carbohydrates can limit the amount of stomach acid that your body produces which is why a lot of athletes have vitamin absorption issues that they are not aware of.

Simple ways to fix poor nutrition absorption

-Eliminate digestive stress by eating less overall food, spacing your meals out more and limiting your exposure to pesticides and chemicals.

-Consider supplementing with Betatine HCL to rebuild your stomach acid.

You're not properly hydrated

When I want to make a athlete perform better almost instantly, I'll put them on a hydration protocol since most athletes walk around dehydrated. Everyone knows that hydration is important, but unless you make a conscience effort to hydrate, you're likely suffering from a certain degree of inadequate fluids. Stop thinking of dehydration in an extreme sense. Just because you're not passing out or having a bad headache doesn't mean that you aren't dehydrated. Just a 2% drop in hydration can significantly impair performance and a 1-1.5 quart loss of water can lead to upwards of a 25% decrease in aerobic endurance. Hydration is also an essential factor for turning on muscle growth.

Simple ways to hyper hydration

-Actively consume an electrolyte beverage. I prefer and recommend the natural Ultima Replenisher.

-Supplement with 5 grams of creatine monohydrate.

You have low testosterone

While I can certainly go deeper about the topic of low testosterone in mixed martial arts (and I do so with my clients), these days athletes face an epidemic of low testosterone. Previous drugs used will have the biggest impact on our current testosterone levels, but other factors such as sleep, chemical exposure, body fat and training affect it as well. Age is not as big of a factor as once thought and there are multiple research studies that support this idea. Environmental toxins and your diet are the two biggest determining factors for anyone looking to get an advantage by increasing their testosterone naturally.

Simple ways to fix low testosterone

-Consume grass fed beef and wild caught salmon at least 5 days per week.

-Eat 3-4 servings of broccoli and kale per day.

-Consider detoxing your body with natural supplements that increase testosterone like DIM and Calcium D Glucarate.

You suffer from micronutrient deficiency

Recovering from training doesn't just depend on what you eat or what type of shake you drink. Identifying and correcting micronutrient deficiencies can greatly impact your performance and physique. Our foods today are just not as enriched with vitamins as they used to be. While it's normal to overlook common nutrient deficiencies in mixed martial artists such as iodine, magnesium, selenium, Vitamin B12 and Vitamin K2, we cannot over look how they impact performance. Lack of muscle recovery, increased muscle fatigue and tearing, fragile bones and increased muscle strains, as well as an overall lack of energy, can negatively impact a training camp to detrimental levels.

Simple ways to fix micronutrient deficiencies

-Rotate the colors of fruits and vegetables that you eat on a daily basis so that you have a wide spectrum of nutrients entering your body.

-Rebuild your stomach acid to increase nutrition absorption.

You have poor sleeping patterns

While reduced insulin sensitivity, high cortisol levels and adrenal fatigue will all negatively impact sleep quality, there are a few other critical factors that can reduce your ability to get a restful night sleep. The main offender is what you eat before you go to bed. When you first enter a deep sleep, your body will release a large growth hormone pulse which both fights fat and helps your body recover from the day's training, unless you ate right before you went to bed. While eating carbohydrates at night isn't a bad idea, eating carbohydrates right before bed is a terrible idea. Doing so will skyrocket your insulin and actually shut off your growth hormone production to a degree.

Eating carbohydrates an hour to two hours before bed will actually cause your body to release more serotonin, a natural brain chemical, so that you can sleep deeper.

Another issue impacting our sleep quality is light in the bedroom from television, cell phones, alarm clocks or street lights. Light exposure, of any kind, causes our biological clock to either speed up or slow down, which affects our sleep and wake cycle. Our ancestors woke up when the sun came up and went to bed shortly after the sun went down. If you're staring at tablet screens or are trying to sleep with an alarm clock in your face, then you're lowering your body's levels of melatonin. Our body produces this sleep hormone to help us relax.

Simple ways to improve your sleep

-Eat a tiny amount of starchy carbohydrates one to two hours before you go to sleep.

-Cover any light in your room and place a towel under your doorway so any light doesn't entire your room.

-Consider supplementing with 200-600 mg's of Magnesium Glycinate one hour before you go to sleep.

You have too much inflammation

In my opinion, the biggest deterrent of your performance is constant inflammation. While there are a number of issues that cause inflammatory responses in your body, the biggest offenders are stress, sugar, too much caffeine, artificial food products, all corn derived products, diary and soy. Chronic inflammation will lower your immune system response, which impacts your training recovery and reduces your ability to gain lean muscle, strength and decreases your endurance.

Simple ways to lower your inflammation

-Consume 6-9 grams of a high quality Omega-3 fish oil supplement daily.

-Eat grass fed beef and wild caught salmon three to four times per week.

-Remove all grains and dairy from your diet for a week then slowly add grains back into your diet.

Your body can't detox properly

Don't think of detoxing as some weird juicing diet or crazy pill based program. Your body can detox itself properly provided that you give it the tools to achieve that goal. Reducing your consumption of non organic meats and farm raised fish is the first step. Unfortunately, we live in a polluted world and just being around someone that smokes or getting stuck in traffic with all the exhaust from cars can greatly impair our ability to detox. We also suffer from increased aromatization due to all the pollution. Aromatization decreases the process where your body purposely lowers your testosterone and turns it into more estrogen and we obviously don't want this.

Simple ways to improve your detox abilities

-Consider using a high quality Calcium D Glucarate and DIM supplement daily.

-Add 1-2 grams of a high quality Curcumin supplement into your diet daily.

-Eat 2-3 servings of broccoli, kale or spinach daily.

The Diet

The goal of this manual is to simplify advanced performance nutrition and I have done that below with meal plan examples for both male and female athletes that will cover all of the issues mentioned above. The goal of this diet is to positively impact your ability to gain strength and lean muscle, improve your VO2 max and burn body fat. This diet is designed for an athlete who needs to compete at 185 pounds. That doesn't mean that someone who has to compete at a lower weight class can't use this approach, they'll just have to lower the carbohydrates. Conversely an athlete who needs to compete in a heavier weight class should likely double the recommended carbohydrate intake.

Meal One: Ideally eaten within 45 minutes of rising.

Pick ONE food option from each listing.

Protein options - PICK ONE
4-6 whole eggs for men
2-4 whole eggs for women

2 cups of cottage cheese or greek yogurt for men
1 cup of cottage cheese or greek yogurt for women

For men: 30 grams of whey protein in 8 ounces of skim milk or almond milk
For women: 20 grams of whey protein in 8 ounces of skim milk or almond milk

4 ounces of bison or grass fed meat for men
2 ounces of bison or grass fed meat for women

For both men and women, one bowl of mixed berries

<u>Fat options - PICK ONE</u>
2-3 pieces of organic bacon for men
1-2 pieces of organic bacon for women

2 tbsp. of extra virgin olive oil for men
1 tbsp. of extra virgin olive oil for women

15 walnuts or almonds or pine nuts for men
12 walnuts or almonds or pine nuts for women

Another option is Jimmy's Super Shake

<u>Jimmy's Super Shake</u>
12 ounces of water
40 grams of vanilla whey protein (women 20 grams of protein)
1/2 cup of frozen blueberries
1/2 cup of frozen strawberries or raspberries (or a mixture of both)
1/2 cup of frozen pineapple

5 grams of creatine monohydrate (optional)
1 cup of plain, non fat, greek yogurt

Add 4-5 ice cubes and blend until you have a smoothie.

<u>Meal Two:</u> This meal is ideal for either a typical lunch or a pre workout meal

PICK ONE OPTION

Option #1
Mixed greens salad with low fat american cheese and 1 medium tomato sliced
For men: 2 handfuls of lean protein, such as salmon, shrimp, chicken or turkey
For women: 1 handful of lean protein, such as salmon, shrimp, chicken or turkey

Option #2
Wrap of your choice with 1 medium tomato sliced with lettuce
For men: 2 handfuls of lean protein, such as tuna, chicken or turkey
For women: 1 handful of lean protein, such as tuna, chicken or turkey

Option #3
Power smoothie
For men:
40 grams of whey protein, 1 cup of greek yogurt, 1 cup of frozen mixed berries and half a

banana mixed with ice cubes and 12 ounces of water and blend until smooth.

For women:

20 grams of whey protein, 1 cup of greek yogurt, 1 cup of frozen mixed berries and a quarter of a banana mixed with ice cubes and 12 ounces of water and blend until smooth.

Option #4: Pro testosterone meal for men
6 ounces of grass fed beef, such as ground beef, top round or sirloin
1/2 cup of almonds, pine nuts or brazil nuts
1 cup of broccoli or kale

Last meal of the evening

Pick ONE food option from each listing
6 ounces of grass fed or organic meat or ground beef for men
3 ounces of grass fed or organic meat or ground beef for women

5 ounces of wild caught salmon or tuna for men
3 ounces of wild caught salmon or tuna for women

6 ounces of organic chicken or turkey for men
4 ounces of organic chicken or turkey for women

Carbohydrate Sources

2 cups of either jasmine, brown or white long grain rice for men
1 cup of either jasmine, brown or white long grain rice for women

1 large sweet or white potato for men
1 small sweet or white potato for women

2 cups of pasta for men
1 cup of pasta for women

4 slices of whole wheat or rye bread for men
2 slices of whole wheat or rye bread for women

Note: You should also eat a large serving of green vegetables with this meal. Your serving should at least fill up your entire palm.

Pre and Post Workout Nutrition

Pre workout meal ideally eaten 60 minutes before your workout.

30 grams of whey mixed with 1 cup of mixed berries

During workout: 5 grams of BCAA's mixed with 2 scoops of Ultima Replenisher

Athletes often get dehydrated even before their body knows it. Ultima Replenisher is a plant based, natural product that rapidly delivers electrolytes without the excessive sugar to working muscles.

<u>Post workout:</u>

For men: 30-40 grams of whey protein isolate in 12 ounces of water with 1 cup of oatmeal or long grain rice or pasta and 1 cup of mixed berries.

For women: 20-25 grams of whey protein isolate in 12 ounces of water with 1/2 cup of oatmeal or long grain rice or pasta and 1 cup of mixed berries.

What to Eat

I understand that the nutrition world can be a crazy place. Diets exist that restrict certain food groups while encouraging large quantities of others. Some diets even label foods as good or bad.

Without getting into it too deeply, there are no good foods or bad foods. Judge your food choices based on your goals and the nutrients that the food provides. While there is never a reason to eliminate any specific food, we want to minimize some foods and maximize our intake of others.

Protein Choices

Chicken (preferably organic)
Beef (preferably grass fed or organic)
Eggs
Milk
Cheese
Tuna
Wild caught fish
Cottage cheese
Greek Yogurt or regular
Turkey
Ham
Pork
Bison
Lamb

Whey protein
Qunioa

Carbohydrate Choices

Oatmeal
White or whole wheat pasta
White or whole wheat bread
White or brown or jasmine rice
White or sweet or red potatoes
Bagels
Berries (blackberries, blueberries, strawberries
or raspberries)
Apples
Avocado
Oranges
Pineapples
Baked potato chips like Pop chips
Organic frozen waffles
Organic popcorn
Beans

Fat Choices

Cheese - white, american, cheddar,
mozzarella, parmesan
Peanut butter
Almond butter
Extra virgin olive oil
Macadamia nut oil
Coconut oil

Ghee or organic butter
Almonds
Walnuts
Pine nuts
Cashews
Pistachios
Brazil Nuts
Omega-3 fish oil supplements

A Note About Vegetables

Vegetables are UNLIMITED and should be consumed with at least 3 meals per day.

Vegetable Choices

Broccoli
Kale
Swiss Chard
Spinach
Green Beans
Asparagus
Collards
Tomatoes
Brussels Sprouts
Carrots
Squash
Sweet Potatoes
Eggplant
Bell Peppers
Onion

Frequently Asked Questions

After seeing the diet, I'm sure that you have some questions. In this section I'm going to address some frequently asked questions in hopes that you'll have a better understanding of why I've designed the meal plan the way that I did.

Isn't eating every 2-3 hours the best way for an athlete to eat?

Absolutely not. As a matter of fact, eating every 2-3 hours doesn't have any positive or special benefits to your performance or physique. While you no doubt have read that you must eat every 2-3 hours to keep your blood sugar levels stable, that information is just rhetoric repeated year after year. The published research on meal frequency has been poorly designed, such as a famous study comparing six solid meals to three liquid meals. No wonder the person that ate six meals felt better, they had more food!

The response that I typically receive is along the lines of people hearing that skipping meals will cause them to gain weight. People often point out sumo wrestlers as an example of why your body stores fat if you don't eat frequently. Those are inaccurate examples. Your body doesn't just flip a switch and turn on any type of fat storing mode because you haven't eaten every few hours. If anything, eating at that pace will more than likely make you hungry.

Your body gets used to incoming levels of foods at specific intervals by ramping up hunger hormones. If you randomly break that schedule, you'll feel lethargic, light headed and hungry. That isn't a good thing. Have you ever been so busy at work that you just didn't have to time to eat? You weren't hungry when you were busy, but the second you sat down you realized that you haven't eaten in a while. Your body didn't break down because you didn't eat nor did you pass out.

By spacing out your meals you gain control over these hunger hormones.

What about the research that says people are likely to gorge after going too long without eating? There are multiple reasons why people gorge on food in general and it's not directly linked to the fact that they don't eat every few hours. There are mental food issues or just an overall lack of focus and commitment to a goal. As a high performance athlete, focus isn't the issue so don't expect to gorge post meal.

Your body only knows the end result of the day. Did you get all of your nutrition in? It doesn't care about the intervals. As a matter of fact, spacing out your meals may have positive benefits on your fat burning, longevity hormones

I heard fasting is bad for my body, should I include it?

Eating is actually very stressful on your body, especially if you're cramming food in every few hours. Digestion is slowed and your body can't properly process all of your food, even if you're eating a perfectly healthy diet. The goal of the Physique Formula is to help you burn fat, build lean muscle, improve your performance, fight inflammation and live healthier. The first benefit that you'll see from eating less overall food and spacing out your meals is increased natural energy.

By spacing your meals further apart, your body will not need to digest as much food as often and it will keep your stress hormones down. Have you ever eaten a meal, even a perfectly good meal, then about 30 minutes later you're tired? This is because your body is raising your stress hormones to process what you just ate.

Another benefit of fasting is that your body will increase its production of human growth hormone. While athletes abuse this drug in high quantities to increase their performance, your body is actually very adept at producing good sized pulses on its own, if you allow it.

Raising your growth hormone will help you recover from training and burn body fat.

I don't include fasting in this plan. However, if you'd like to start, simply wait a few hours after you wake up on an off training day and try it. You're allowed to drink coffee, tea or water during the fast. Start by spacing out your meals a little more infrequently like I recommend.

If you want more guidance on fasting, email me at jimmy@jimmysmithtraining.com.

Should I avoid eating fat and carbohydrates together?

This is another old theory in nutrition that has no place in the nutrition plan of high level athletes. The theory used to be that eating a fat based food like nuts with a carbohydrate based food like rice or in an extreme example, pizza, would set your body up for fat storage. That's inaccurate. Each food group (protein, fat and carbohydrates) has their own unique benefits and down side. Following the plans that I designed will give your body the right nutrients in the right quantities at the right time.

I've been told that I need to eat 2 grams of protein per pound of body weight to gain muscle, is this true?

That's complete overkill. Eating large quantities of protein will not cause your body to build bigger muscles or get stronger quicker than someone who eats less. In research, the term high protein actually means only about .7-.8 grams of protein per pound of body weight. When you're eating close to 2 grams of protein, your body eventually burns that extra protein for energy, which is not what you want. You want your body to use stored body fat for energy. As long as hard training athletes reach their protein limit with each meal, they'll top out their protein needs during the course of the day. A hard training athlete only needs about 1 gram of protein per pound of body weight.

A guy at my gym uses a gluten free paleo diet, isn't that better than your diet?

When you break down the paleo diet versus The Physique Formula you'll see that they are almost identical with one difference, I include starchy carbohydrates. While the paleo diet is a good approach and I'm sure the person at your gym thinks it's fantastic, it's not ideal for hard training athletes.

When you limit starchy carbohydrates in a hard training athlete diet you'll impair that athlete's recovery. Training raises the stress hormone cortisol which breaks down lean muscle. When cortisol is high the hard training athlete will never recover from training properly. Recovery is also dependent on muscle glycogen, which is how your body stores the starchy carbohydrates that you eat. You'll never fill your glycogen stores by eating just fruits and vegetables.

The relatively small amount of carbohydrates that The Physique Formula recommends won't wreck your gut health or make you fat or reduce your longevity. It'll just make you a better, leaner athlete.

My friend is a vegan and says that I'd feel better and live longer if I didn't eat meat. Is that true?

That is completely inaccurate and while I'm sure that there are athletes who are vegan and swear by it, they are confused. I'll agree that commercially raised animal products are not good for us. Animals are fed large amounts of hormones and corn, which are bad for them and us. When your friend cut all animal products out of their diet, they probably immediately felt better but what else did they switch? Did they finally cut sugar or caffeine out too? Did they finally start eating more fruits, vegetables and fish? Did they stop smoking, drinking or finally sleep more?

Do you see my point? There are numerous variables that determine how good a vegan feels independently of their lack of meat.

Plus, The Physique Formula only advocates grass fed or organic meat, beef, chicken, turkey or lamb and wild caught fish. These sources are free of hormones, corn or pesticides.

Should I stop eating carbohydrates after 5 or 6 at night, right?

This is another old theory that refuses to go away. Your metabolism isn't higher in the morning and lower at night. Your body doesn't work in any set pattern and your metabolism is dictated by your height, weight, age, muscle mass, body fat and activity level. If you overeat carbohydrates day after day, that's when you'll gain weight. Your carbohydrate limits are set to fuel your activity while helping you drop body fat. Plus, eating carbohydrates later in the day has numerous benefits. You won't experience any type of energy crash earlier in the day because your blood sugar will be stabilized with your protein and fat based meals. Carbohydrates eaten at night time actually help your body produce more of the relaxation chemical serotonin which will help you sleep better. Your night time growth hormone levels will also get a nice nighttime bump from carbohydrates eaten before bed, as well for increased fat loss and longevity.

My old nutritionist told me that I should only eat certain foods on a diet, is that true?

For starters, this is a nutrition plan not a diet. A diet implies that this is a short term fix, The Physique Formula isn't that. There are no good diet foods and there are no bad diet foods. There are certainly some foods that are better than others. Your body only recognizes the protein, carbohydrates and fats in any food source. Your body will handle the carbohydrates in a candy bar or cookie in the exact same way that it will handle the carbohydrates in rice or oatmeal. Now I'm not advising you to eat a candy bar every day, I'm merely pointing out that you have access to a greater variety of food than you think.

Recent studies examine white rice versus brown rice in people attempting to lose body fat. The results? Both groups lost exactly the same amount of weight.

At the end of the day, all that matters, is that you provide your body with the proper amount of macronutrients (protein, carbohydrates and fats) and micronutrients (the vitamins in food) that it needs and you will achieve results.

Should I have a post workout shake?

This is where I'm going to make some enemies. A whey protein shake after an intense training session is a fantastic idea in order to speed muscle recovery. A shake containing whey protein and any sort of fast acting carbohydrate like waxy maize or dextrose isn't the best. Why? For starters, waxy maize and dextrose are corn based products and the human digestive system has an extreme sensitivity to corn. Plus, these drinks are sugar based.

The idea that you need sugar immediately post workout is out dated and frankly, a terrible recommendation. Why would I want to ingest 30 or 40 grams of sugar and spike my blood sugar? It's not for recovery because sugar doesn't aid in recovery. The only exception being if an athlete was doing back to back training sessions, like in mixed martial arts or track and field where an athlete does a weight workout then shortly after a technique workout. If your training sessions are spread apart by a few hours, a solid carbohydrate meal will do just fine for increasing recovery and it's good for your health, which is just a little important as well.

Bonus Checklist: How To Cut Weight Safely and Effectively Rehydrate

Since I know that a majority of the athletes who will read this manual will, at some point, have to cut weight in order to meet a weight class requirement, I wanted to include this simple checklist so that twenty four to forty eight hours before the weight cut can be as painless and effortless at possible.

I've worked with multiple elite mixed martial artists and I've seen the good, bad and the ugly of the weight cut. Honestly, I've seen fighters take risks that they didn't have to, but they do so because they assume it's the best approach. In reality, there are simple and effective ways for losing upward of fifteen to twenty pounds in a matter of hours safely.

Step One: Make sure that you've actually set goals with your diet before the weight cut.
There's nothing worse than an athlete who is attempting to cut upwards of twenty five pounds a day or two before a fight. The diet leading up to the competition should be goal oriented and leave you within ten to fifteen pounds of your competition weight.

Step Two: Don't run or exercise to attempt to dehydrate and get rid of excessive water underneath the skin.

Any type of muscular effort close to the competition will place an extreme strain on your central nervous system which will limit your potential force production during your competition. Maybe it has worked for you in the past, but you can do better.

Step Three: Eliminating water and sodium too soon.

Your body tightly regulates intra cellular fluid volume. Eliminating water and sodium too soon before a weight cut causes your body to release the water storing hormone, aldosterone. Your body senses that it doesn't know when it's going to get water again so it closely maintains its current fluid volume. Then the cycle starts again. The athlete will sit in a sauna or go for another jog, which further reduces the potential force that they can produce later on.

Step Four: Don't use the sauna to cut weight.

Sitting in the sauna will expose you to dry heat. Your body won't flush out as much water since your body won't sweat in order to cool your core temperature. A sauna is dry heat which just prolongs the duration of the hard cut.

Step Five: Sleep in a cold room.

After you've performed your traditional weight cut you should sleep in a cold room. Your body will still have a high core temperature and will attempt to cool itself off during the course of the night resulting in a lower bodyweight when you wake up.

Step Six: Don't cut all the weight at once.
You want to cut weight slowly over the course of about thirty six hours. Doing this reduces the impact on your muscular and central nervous systems which will help you to maintain your force production during the competition. You'll also rehydrate easier.

Step Seven: Drinking the wrong thing after the weigh-in.
I cringe every time I see a high level athlete drinking a popular sports drink when they step off the scale. These drinks contain too much sugar which slows down the absorption of the nutrients in the drink by the small intestine. The sugar in the drink defeats the purpose of the drink in the first place! That's not to say that athletes shouldn't rehydrate once they step off the scale, they just need to do it properly.

Step Eight: Too much, too soon.
I understand that the meal post weight cut can be the most satisfying reward but athletes often wreck their chances of success because they eat too quickly. After a weight cut your body is a sponge and can absorb and store food at a rapid rate. Just sitting down and eating isn't enough. An athlete must take specific supplements to increase nutrient absorption.

For customized weight cutting services email Jimmy directly at
jimmy@jimmysmithtraining.com

Bonus Checklist: How To Reverse "Permanent" Joint Pain

I use the word "permanent" very loosely. Often times, in my experience, athletes who suffer career threatening injuries most often do NOT need to go under the knife and have surgery. Sure, there are specific cases like ACL tears and the like, but more often than not a serious joint injury is a result of an improper movement pattern leading to faulty joint mechanics that eventually fail during a high intensity activity.

Using the following checklist will minimize inflammation that is running rampant in the your body. Inflammation isn't a bad thing except when it's excessive.

Step One: Identify any potential food sensitivities and remove the offenders from your diet.
An estimated 45-60% of the population suffers from some form of undiagnosed food sensitivity symptoms that are impacting recovery, breaking down joints and wrecking your immune system health. After you consume a potentially sensitive ingredient your body

36

ramps up its production of IgE, an antibody that tags the food as a foreign invader. If you have a sensitivity to a certain food that you ate, then a whole variety of potential reactions can occur, including gastrointestinal tract discomfort, bloating, diarrhea, mucus formation and itchy skin, as well as nerve based pain such as tingling or the feeling of pins and needles.

Some of the more common foods known to cause minor to severe reactions include yeast, lactose, gluten, fructose, food preservatives and nitrates, amines found in cheese and pickles, salicylates found in nuts, soy sauce and jams, monosodium glutamate found in processed food and Chinese food and propionates found in commercial bread.

I cannot stress enough that minor food sensitivities may not cause any reaction at all, but that does not mean that you are not being negatively impacted by a sensitivity.

Step Two: Begin using andrographolides supplements.

This has nothing to do with the hormone substance andro. They are completely different molecules and andrographolides will have no impact on your hormone levels. Research has shown that andrographolides has the unique ability to both reduce the tenderness and swelling of a joint, as well reduce the perceived pain caused by the injured joint.

Step Three: Increase your Curcumin dosage.

I discussed Curcumin in the "*Your body can't detox*" section above, but this unique spice also has powerful anti-inflammatory properties. The reason that joints seem to slowly breakdown a tiny bit more month after month is a result of an increased gene expression known as matrix metalloproteinases (MMP). Think of MMP as a wrecking ball that slowly erodes away cartilage. Research shows that Curcumin may potentially block this pathway resulting in less joint pain.

Step Four: Prolotherapy.

This increasingly popular cocktail injection works by increasing the number of collagen fibers in order to bring blood to the injured or painful area and stimulate new tissue growth. The Mayo Clinic reports that the joints most likely to benefit from this treatment are the knees, elbows, ankles and low back.

Step Five: Platelet Rich Plasma (PRP).

The most popular choice for today's elite athlete is PRP treatment which involves the plasma found in every ounce of your blood. As the platelets are drawn out of your body, they are then compounded with growth and healing factors. These natural growth and healing factors are then spun in a centrifuge with separates red blood cells from the platelets. They are then injected back into the body and release certain healing enzymes which regenerate ligament and tendon fibers.

The act of PRP itself is 100% legal, but some athletes do choose to take further steps and have growth factors added into the treatment. I do not recommend this step at all and any athlete that chooses to do this may not pass a drug test.

Bonus: How To Recover From Brain Trauma

The topic of concussions in sports has been a hot discussion lately and with good reason. What often gets ignored, however, is the brain trauma that isn't a diagnosed concussion. The repeated head strikes in mixed martial arts or the jarring from a kneeling stance in football often result in head trauma that never results in a concussion so the athlete is never treated. Just because every blow doesn't result in concussion like symptoms doesn't mean that it's not something that we should be concerned about.

Neuroscientist Daniel G.Amen MD was the lead researcher on a recently published study in the *Journal of Psychoactive Drugs* titled "Reversing Brain Damage in Former NFL Players". The surprising thing about the study was that the subjects, eight former NFL players, did not use drugs, instead they used nutritional supplements to improve their brain health after repeated trauma. After six months of using a protocol similar to what I am going to describe below, some of the athletes showed upwards of 50% improvement in brain health.

Anyone that has suffered from repeated blows to the head would be best served to employ the following nutrition tactics.

- Add a larger amount of high quality fat from sources such as high dose Omega-3 fish oil, almonds, pine nuts and extra virgin olive oil. Fats are needed for proper brain cell health and communication.
- Consume two to three cups or green tea per day. Research has shown that green tea has numerous positive benefits for reducing brain inflammation.
- Ensure nightly adequate sleep.
- Limit alcohol and cigarette use.
- Consider supplementing with the nutrient vinopocetine. Used as a drug in Eastern Europe for the treatment of age related memory loss, vinpocetine has been shown to enhance brain blood flow and reduce inflammation in addition to displaying numerous neuroprotective effects.
- Being using a phosphatidylserine supplement. This fat soluble nutrient is one of the more effective brain health supplements that you can take. Studies have shown that supplementing with phosphatidylserine improves memory and cognition, as well as enhancing sports performance by decreasing muscle damage and lowering the hormonal response to stress. It has also been shown to be a proven mood enhancer.

Conclusion

My goal in writing this book is to help you, the athlete, perform better and live a leaner and healthier life. I hope that I was able to better educate you on nutrition and give you an easier path to success.

Obviously, space was limited and there was no way that I could include all of the advanced nutritional techniques and methods that I use with my clients. As a result, I'm offering a special consultation to any athlete that reads this manual and emails me directly at jimmy@jimmysmithtraining.com with the headline "Athlete Consultation".

Expect Greatness!

Jimmy Smith,MS,CSCS
www.jimmysmithtraining.com